The Ultimate
Healthy Instant Pot
Cookbook 2021

Quick and Easy Instant Pot Recipes to Enjoy
Everyday Life and Cook Nutritious Tasty Meals
for Stay Healthy!

Brenda Cole

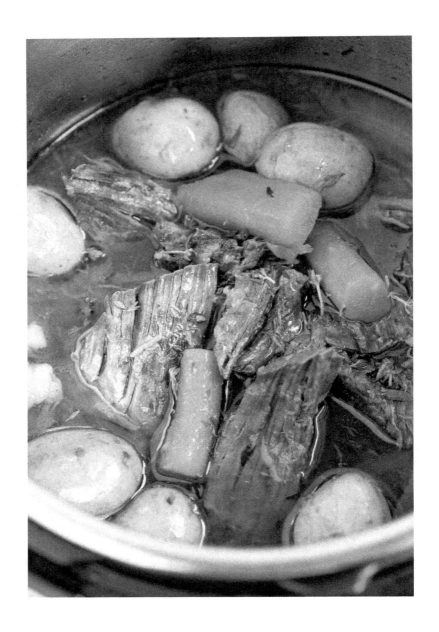

Table of Contents

solely under their purview. There are no scenarios in which the publisher or the original author of this work can be in any fashion deemed liable for any hardship or damages that may befall them after undertaking information described herein. Additionally, the information in the following pages is intended only for informational purposes and should thus be thought of as universal. As befitting its nature, it is presented without assurance regarding its prolonged validity or interim quality. Trademarks that are mentioned are done without written consent and can in no way be considered an endorsement from the trademark holder.

Introduction

Instant pot is a pressure cooker, also stir-fry, stew, and cook rice, cook vegetables and chicken. It's an all-in-one device, so you can season chicken and cook it in the same pan, for example. In most cases, instant pot meals can be served in less than an hour.

Cooking less time is due to the pressure cooking function that captures the steam generated by the liquid cooking environment (including liquids released from meat and vegetables), boosts the pressure and pushes the steam back.

But don't confuse with traditional pressure cookers. The instant pot, unlike the pressure cooker used by grandparents, eliminates the risk of safety with a lid that locks and remains locked until pressure is released.

Even when cooking time is over in the instant pot, you need to take an additional step-to release the pressure.

There are two ways to relieve pressure. Due to the natural pressure release, the lid valve remains in the sealing position and the pressure will naturally dissipate over time. This process takes 20 minutes to over an hour, depending on what is cooked. Low fluidity foods (such as chicken wings) take less time than high fluidity foods such as soups and marinades.

Another option is manual pressure release (also called quick release). Now you need to carefully move the valve to the ventilation position and see that the steam rises slowly and the pressure is released. This Directions is much faster, but foods with high liquid content, such as soups, take about 15 minutes to manually relieve pressure.

Which option should I use? Take into account that even if natural pressure is released, the instant pot is still under pressure. This means that the food will continue to cook while the instant pot is in sealed mode. Manual pressure relief is useful when the dishes are well cooked and need to be stopped as soon as possible.

If the goal is to prepare meals quickly, set the cooking time for dishes that are being cooked in an instant pop and release the pressure manually after the time has passed.

Instant pots (called "Instapot" by many) are one of our favorite cookware because they can handle such a wide range of foods almost easily. Instant pots range from those that work on the basics of pressure cooking to those that can be sterilized using Suicide video or some models can be controlled via Wi-Fi.

In addition, if you want to expand the range of kitchenware, the Instant Pot brand has released an air fryer that can be used to make rotisserie chicken and homemade beef jerky. There is also an independent accumulator device that can be used in instant pots to make fish, steaks and more.

The current icon instant pot works like a pressure cooker and uses heat and steam to quickly cook food. Everything from perfect carnitas to boiled eggs was cooked, but not all ingredients and DIRECTIONSs work. Here are few foods that should not be cooked in classic instant pots.

Instant pots are not pressure fryer and are not designed to handle the high temperatures required to heat cooking oils like crispy fried chicken. Of course, the instant pot is great for dishes like Carnitas, but after removing the meat from the instant pot, to get the final crispness in the meat, transfer it to a frying pan for a few minutes or to an oven top and hot Crispy in the oven.

As with slow cookers, dairy products such as cheese, milk, and sour cream will pack into instant pots using pressure cooking settings or slow cooking settings. Do not add these ingredients after the dish are cooked or create a recipe in Instapot.

There are two exceptions. One is when making yogurt. This is merely possible if you are using an instant pot recipe. The other is only when making cheesecake and following an instant pot recipe.

Although you can technically cook pasta in an instant pot, gummy may appear and cooking may be uneven. To be honest, unless you have a choice, cooking pasta in a stove pot is just as fast and easy and consistently gives you better cooked pasta.

Instead of baking the cake in an instant pot, steam it. The cake is moist-it works for things like bread pudding-but there is no good skin on the cake or on the crunchy edge everyone fights with a baked brownie. However, let's say your desire is to build a close-up or a simple dessert with your family; you can get a damp sponge in about 30 minutes, except during the DIRECTIONS time.

Canning, a technique for cooking and sealing food in a jar, is often done in a pressure cooker. Therefore, it is recommended to create a batch of jam, pickles or jelly in Instapot. Please do not.

With an instant pot, you can't monitor the temperature of what you can, like a normal pressure cooker. In canning, it is important to cook and seal the dishes correctly. Incorrect cooking and sealing can lead to the growth of bacteria that can cause food poisoning.

If you want to avoid canning in an instant pot, some newer models, such as Duo Plus, have a sterilization setting that can clean kitchen items such as baby bottles, bottles and cookware.

Instant Pot Pressure Cooker Safety Tips

Instant Pot is a very safe pressure cooker consisting of various safety mechanisms. do not worry. It will not explode immediately. Most accidents are caused by user errors and can be easily avoided. To further minimize the possibility of an accident, we have compiled a list of safety tips.

1 Don't leave it alone

It is not recommended to leave home while cooking an instant pot. If you have to leave it alone, make sure it is under pressure and no steam is coming out.

2 Do not use KFC in instant pot

Do not fry in an instant pot or other pressure cooker.

KFC uses a commercial pressure fryer specially made to fry chicken (the latest one that operates at 5 PSI). Instant pots (10.5-11.6 PSI) are specially made to make our lives easier.

3 water intake!

Instant pots require a minimum of 1 1/2 cup liquid (Instant Pot Official Number) 1 cup liquid to reach and maintain pressure.

The liquid can be a combination of gravy, vinegar, water, chicken etc.

4 half full or half empty

The max line printed on the inner pot of the instant pot is not for pressure cooking.

For pressure cooking: up to 2/3 full

Food for pressure cooking that expands during cooking (grains, beans, dried vegetables, etc.): up to 1/2

5 Not a facial steamer

Deep cleaning is not performed even if the pressure cooker steam is used once.

When opening, always tilt the lid away from you. Wear waterproof and heat-resistant silicone gloves especially when performing quick release.

6 never use power

In situations of zero, you should try to force open the lid of the instant pot pressure cooker, unless you want to prevent a light saber from hitting your face.

7 Wash Up & Checkout

If you want to be secured, wash the lid after each use and clean the anti-block shield and inner pot. Make sure that the gasket (silicon seal ring) is in good shape and that there is no food residue in the anti-block shield before use.

Usually silicone seal rings should be replaced every 18-24 months. It is always advisable to keep extra things.

Do not purchase a sealing ring from a third party because it is an integral part of the safety features of the instant ring. Using sealing rings that have not been tested with instant pot products can create serious safety concerns."

Before use, make sure that the sealing ring is securely fixed to the sealing ring rack and the anti-block shield is properly attached to the vapor discharge pipe.

A properly fitted sealing ring can be moved clockwise or counterclockwise in the sealing ring rack with little force.

With instant pots, the whole family can cook meals in less than 30 minutes. Cooked dishes such as rice, chicken, beef stew, sauce, yakitori can be cooked for 30-60 minutes from the beginning to the end. And yes, you can bake bread in an instant pot.

Old and ketogenic diet fans love instant pots for their ability to `` roast " meat in such a short time, but vegetarians and vegans that can quickly cook dishes such as pumpkin soup, baked potatoes and marinated potato chilis, also highly appreciated oatmeal cream and macaroni and cheese.

Even dried beans, which usually require overnight cooking, can be prepared in 30 minutes to make spicy hummus.

Coconut Chicken and Peppers

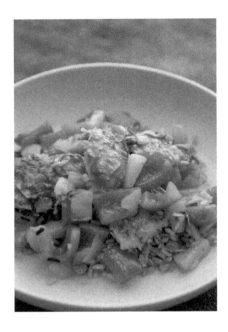

Preparation Time: 10 minutes

Cooking Time: 24 minutes

Servings: 4

Ingredients:

1 cup chicken stock

A pinch of salt and black pepper

1 pound chicken breast, skinless, boneless and cubed

1 tablespoon coconut, unsweetened and shredded

1 tablespoon oregano, chopped

½ pound mixed peppers, cut into strips

1 tablespoon chives, chopped

1 tablespoon olive oil

Directions:

Put your instant pot on Sauté mode, add the oil, heat it up, add the onion and the chicken and brown for 2 minutes on each side.

Add the rest of the ingredients, close it and cook on High for 20 minutes.

Naturally release the pressure for 10 minutes, divide everything between plates then serve.

Nutrition:
Protein – 33.2 g.

Calories – 256

Fat – 12.6 g.

Carbs – 1.2 g.

Basil Chili Chicken

Preparation Time: 5 minutes

Cooking Time: 24 minutes

Servings: 4

Ingredients:

1 pound chicken breast, skinless, boneless and cubed

A pinch of salt and black pepper

1 tablespoon chili powder

1 cup coconut cream

2 teaspoons sweet paprika

½ cup chicken stock

2 tablespoons basil, chopped

Directions:

In your instant pot, combine the chicken with the rest of the ingredients,   toss a bit, close it and cook on High for 24 minutes.

Naturally release the pressure for 10 minutes, divide the mix between plates and serve.

Nutrition:

Calories – 364

Protein – 35.4 g.

Fat – 23.2 g.

Carbs – 5.1 g.

Chicken and Oregano Sauce

Preparation Time: 10 minutes

Cooking Time: 20 minutes

Servings: 4

Ingredients:

2 chicken breasts, skinless, boneless and halved

1 tablespoon lemon juice

2 tablespoons olive oil

2 tablespoons oregano, chopped

1 cup tomato passata

1 teaspoon ginger, grated

Directions:

Put the instant pot on Sauté mode, add the oil, heat it up, add tomato passata and remaining ingredients except the chicken, whisk and cook for 5 minutes.

Add the chicken, close and cook on High for 15 minutes. Naturally release the pressure for 10 minutes, divide the mix between plates and serve.

Nutrition:

Calories – 300

Protein – 33.9 g.

Fat – 15.8 g.

Carbs – 5.2 g.

Balsamic Curry Chicken

Preparation Time: 10 minutes

Cooking Time: 20 minutes

Servings: 4

Ingredients:

1 pound chicken breast, skinless, boneless and cubed

A pinch of salt and black pepper

1 cup chicken stock

1 cup coconut cream

3 garlic cloves, minced

1 and ½ tablespoon balsamic vinegar

1 tablespoon chives, chopped

Directions:

In your instant pot, combine the chicken with the rest of the ingredients, close it and cook on High for 20 minutes. Naturally release the pressure for 10 minutes, divide the mix between plates and serve.

Nutrition:

Calories – 360

Protein – 34.5 g.

Fat – 22.1 g.

Carbs – 4.3 g.

Chicken and Eggplant Mix

Preparation Time: 10 minutes

Cooking Time: 20 minutes

Servings: 4

Ingredients:

2 chicken breasts, skinless, boneless and halved

A pinch of salt and black pepper

2 eggplants, roughly cubed

2 tablespoons olive oil

1 cup tomato passata

1 tablespoon oregano, dried

Directions:

In your instant pot, combine all the ingredients, close it and cook on High for 20 minutes.

Naturally release the pressure for 10 minutes, divide between plates and serve.

Nutrition:

Calories – 362

Protein – 36.4 g.

Fat – 16.1 g.

Carbs – 5.4 g.

Sesame Chicken

Preparation Time: 10 minutes

Cooking Time: 20 minutes

Servings: 4

Ingredients:

2 chicken breasts, skinless, boneless and cubed

A pinch of salt and black pepper

1 teaspoon sesame seeds

4 garlic cloves, minced

1 cup tomato passata

1 tablespoon parsley, chopped

1 tablespoon oregano, chopped

Directions:

In your instant pot, mix all the ingredients except the sesame seeds, close it and cook on High for 20 minutes. Naturally release the pressure for 10 minutes, divide everything between plates and serve with the sesame seeds sprinkled on top.

Nutrition:

Calories – 243

Protein – 34.1 g.

Fat – 9 g.

Carbs – 5.4 g.

Turkey and Spring Onions Mix

Preparation Time: 10 minutes

Cooking Time: 25 minutes

Servings: 4

Ingredients:

1 turkey breast, skinless, boneless and cubed

2 tablespoons avocado oil

salt and black pepper

4 spring onions, chopped

1 cup tomato passata

A handful cilantro, chopped

Directions:

Put your instant pot on Sauté mode, add the oil, heat it up, add the meat and brown for 5 minutes.

Add the rest of the ingredients, close it and cook on High for 20 minutes.

Naturally release the pressure for 10 minutes between plates, divide the turkey mix between plates, and serve.

Nutrition:

Calories – 222

Protein – 34.4 g.

Fat – 6.7 g.

Carbs – 4.8 g.

Italian Paprika Chicken

Preparation Time: 10 minutes

Cooking Time: 20 minutes

Servings: 4

Ingredients:

1 pound chicken breasts, skinless, boneless and cubed

A pinch of salt and black pepper

1 tablespoon olive oil

1 tablespoon sweet paprika

1 tablespoon Italian seasoning

2 garlic cloves, minced

1 and ½ cups chicken stock

Directions:

Put your instant pot on Sauté mode, add the oil, heat it up, add the meat and brown for 5 minutes.

Add the rest of the ingredients, close it and cook on High for 15 minutes.

Naturally release the pressure for 10 minutes, divide between plates and serve.

Nutrition:

Calories – 264

Protein – 33.2 g.

Fat – 13.2 g. ,Carbs – 1.9 g.

Tomato Turkey and Sprouts

Preparation Time: 10 minutes

Cooking Time: 25 minutes

Servings: 4

Ingredients:

1 big turkey breast, skinless, boneless and cubed

1 tablespoon avocado oil

1 pound Brussels sprouts

1 teaspoon chili powder

salt and black pepper

1 and ½ cups tomato passata

2 tablespoons cilantro, chopped

Directions:

Put the instant poton Sauté mode, add the oil, heat it up, add the meat and brown for 5 minutes.

Add the rest of the ingredients, close it and cook on High for 20 minutes.

Naturally release the pressure for 10 minutes, divide the mix between plates and serve.

Nutrition:

Protein – 37.3 g., Calories – 249,Fat – 6.6 g. ,Carbs – 4.5 g.

Chicken and Sage Scallops

Preparation Time: 5 minutes

Cooking Time: 10 minutes

Servings: 4

Ingredients:

4 skinless chicken breasts

2 and ½ ounces almond meal

1-ounce parmesan, grated

6 sage leaves, chopped

1 and ¾ ounces almond flour

2 eggs, beaten

Directions:

Take cling paper and wrap chicken with cling wrap
Beat into ½ cm thickness using a rolling pin

Take separate bowls add parmesan, sage, almond meal, flour and beaten eggs into the different bowls

Take chicken and dredge into flour, eggs, breadcrumbs and finally parmesan

Pre-heat your Fryer to 392 degrees F

Take the basket out and spray chicken with oil on both sides

Cook chicken for 5 minutes each side until golden

Serve and enjoy!

Nutrition:

Calories: 264

Fat: 18g

Carbohydrates: 3g

Protein: 19g

Cool Cheese Dredged Chicken

Preparation Time: 10 minutes

Cooking Time: 10 minutes

Servings: 4

Ingredients:

2-piece (6 ounces each) chicken breast, fat trimmed and sliced up in half

6 tablespoons seasoned breadcrumbs

2 tablespoons parmesan, grated

1 tablespoon melted butter

2 tablespoons low-fat mozzarella cheese

½ cup marinara sauce

Cooking spray as needed

Directions:

Pre-heat your Air Fryer to 390-degree Fahrenheit for about 9 minutes

Take the cooking basket and spray it evenly with cooking spray

Take a small bowl and add breadcrumbs and parmesan cheese

Mix them well

Take another bowl and add the butter, melt it in your microwave

Brush the chicken pieces with the butter and dredge them into the breadcrumb mix

Once the fryer is ready, place 2 pieces of your prepared chicken breast and spray the top a bit of oil

Cook for about 6 minutes

Turn them over and top them up with 1 tablespoon of Marinara and 1 and a ½ tablespoon of shredded mozzarella

Cook for 3 minutes more until the cheese has completely melted

Keep the cooked breasts on the side and repeat with the remaining pieces

Nutrition:

Calories: 244

Fat: 14g

Carbohydrates: 15g

Protein: 12g

Spiced Up Air Fried Buffalo Wings

Preparation Time: 10 minutes

Cooking Time: 30 minutes

Servings: 4

Ingredients:

4 pounds chicken wings

½ cup cayenne pepper sauce

½ cup coconut oil

1 tablespoon Worcestershire sauce

1 teaspoon salt

Directions:

Take a mixing cup and add cayenne pepper sauce, coconut oil, Worcestershire sauce and salt
Mix well and keep it on the side
Pat the chicken dry and transfer to your fryer

Cook for 25 minutes at 380-degree F, making sure to shake the basket once

Increase the temperature to 400-degree F and cook for 5 minutes more

Remove them and dump into a large sized mixing bowl

Add the prepared sauce and toss well

Serve with celery sticks and enjoy!

Nutrition:

Calories: 244

Fat: 20g

Carbohydrates: 6g

Protein: 8g

Creamy Onion Chicken

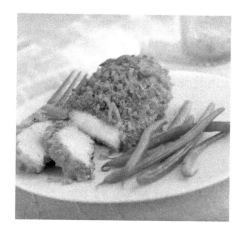

Preparation Time: 30 minutes

Cooking Time: 30 minutes

Servings: 4

Ingredients:

4 chicken breasts

1 and ½ cup onion soup mix

1 cup mushroom soup

½ cup cream

Directions:

Pre-heat your Fryer to 400-degree F.

Take a frying pan and place it over low heat.

Add mushrooms, onion mix and cream.

Heat up the mixture for 1 minute.

Pour the warm mixture over chicken and let it sit for 25 minutes.

Transfer your marinade chicken to Air Fryer cooking basket and cook for 30 minutes.

Serve with remaining cream and enjoy!

Nutrition:

Calories: 282

Fat: 4g

Carbohydrates: 55g

Protein: 8g

Baked Coconut Chicken

Preparation Time: 5 minutes

Cooking Time: 12 minutes

Servings: 6

Ingredients:

2 large eggs

2 teaspoons garlic powder

1 teaspoon salt

1/2 teaspoon ground black pepper

¾ cup coconut amino

¾ cup shredded coconut

1-pound chicken tenders

Cooking spray

Directions:

Pre-heat your fryer to 400-degree Fahrenheit.

Take a large sized baking sheet and spray it with cooking spray.

Take a wide dish and add garlic powder, eggs, pepper and salt.

Whisk well until everything is combined.

Add the almond meal and coconut and mix well.

Take your chicken tenders and dip them in egg followed by dipping in the coconut mix.

Shake off any excess.

Transfer them to your fryer and spray the tenders with a bit of oil.

Cook for 12-14 minutes until you have a nice golden-brown texture.

Enjoy!

Nutrition:

Calories: 175

Fat: 1g

Carbohydrates: 3g

Protein: 0g

Lemon Pepper Chicken

Preparation Time: 3 minutes

Cooking Time: 15 minutes

Servings: 2

Ingredients:

1 chicken breast

2 lemon, juiced and rind reserved

1 tablespoon chicken seasoning

1 teaspoon garlic puree

Handful of peppercorns

Salt and pepper to taste

Directions:

Pre-heat your fryer to 352-degree F.
Take a large sized sheet of silver foil and work on top,
add all of the seasoning alongside the lemon rind.

Lay out the chicken breast onto a chopping board and trim any fat and little bones.

Season each side with the pepper and salt.

Rub the chicken seasoning on both sides well.

Place on your silver foil sheet and rub.

Seal it up tightly.

Slap it with rolling pin and flatten it.

Place it in your fryer and cook for 15 minutes until the center is fully cooked.

Serve and enjoy!

Nutrition:

Calories: 301

Fat: 22g

Carbohydrates: 11g

Protein: 23g

Crunchy Mustard Chicken

Preparation Time: 20 minutes

Cooking Time: 50 minutes

Servings: 4

Ingredients:

4 garlic cloves

8 chicken slices

1 tablespoon thyme leaves

½ cup dry wine vinegar

Salt as needed

½ cup Dijon mustard

2 cups almond meal

2 tablespoons melted butter

1 tablespoon lemon zest

2 tablespoons olive oil

Directions:

Pre-heat your Air Fryer to 350-degree F

Take a bowl and add garlic, salt, cloves, almond meal, pepper, olive oil, melted butter and lemon zest

Take another bowl and mix mustard and wine

Place chicken slices in the wine mixture and then in the crumb mixture

Transfer prepared chicken to your Air Fryer cooking basket and cook for 40 minutes.

Serve and enjoy!

Nutrition:

Calories: 762

Fat: 24g

Carbohydrates: 3g

Protein: 76g

Caprese Chicken with Balsamic Sauce

Preparation Time: 5 minutes

Cooking Time: 25 minutes

Servings: 6

Ingredients:

 6 chicken breasts

6 basil leaves

¼ cup balsamic vinegar

6 slices tomato

1 tablespoon butter

6 slices mozzarella cheese

Directions:

Pre-heat your Fryer to 400-degree F.

Take a frying and place it over medium heat, add butter and balsamic vinegar and let it melt.

Cover the chicken meat with the marinade.

Transfer chicken to your Air Fryer cooking basket and cook for 20 minutes.

Cover cooked chicken with basil, tomato slices and cheese.

Serve and enjoy!

Nutrition:

Calories: 740
Fat: 54g
Carbohydrates: 4g
Protein: 30g

Grilled Hawaiian Chicken

Preparation Time: 10 minutes

Cooking Time: 15 minutes

Servings: 2

Ingredients:

4 chicken breasts

2 garlic cloves

½ cup ketchup, Keto-friendly

½ teaspoon ginger

½ cup coconut amino

2 tablespoons red wine vinegar

½ cup pineapple juice

2 tablespoons apple cider vinegar

Directions:

Pre-heat your Air Fryer to 360-degree F.

Take a bowl and mix in ketchup, pineapple juice, cider vinegar, ginger.

Take a frying and place it over low heat, add sauce and let it heat up.

Cover chicken with the amino and vinegar, pour hot sauce on top.

Let the chicken sit for 15 minutes to marinade.

Transfer chicken to your Air Fryer and bake for 15 minutes.

Serve and enjoy!

Nutrition:

Calories: 200

Fat: 3g

Carbohydrates: 10g

Protein: 29g

Air Fryer Roasted Garlic Chicken

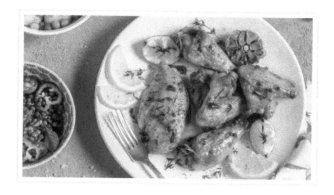

Preparation Time: 5 minutes

Cooking Time: 50 minutes

Servings: 16

Ingredients

4 pounds whole chicken

4 cloves of garlic, minced

Salt and pepper to taste

Directions

Preheat the air fryer at 3300F for 5 minutes

Season the whole chicken with garlic, salt, and pepper.

Place in the air fryer basket.

Cook for 30 minutes at 3300F.

Flip the chicken on the other side and cook for another 20 minutes.

Serve and enjoy!

Nutrition:

Calories: 282

Fat: 4g

Carbohydrates: 55g

Protein: 8g

Air Fried Chicken

Preparation Time: 5 minutes

Cooking Time: 30 minutes

Serves: 4

Ingredients

1 large egg, beaten

¼ cup coconut milk

4 small chicken thighs

½ cup almond flour

1 tablespoon old bay Cajun seasoning

Salt and pepper to taste

Directions

Preheat the air fryer at 3500F for 5 minutes.

Mix the egg and coconut milk in a bowl.

Soak the chicken thighs in the beaten egg mixture.

In a mixing bowl, combine the almond flour, Cajun seasoning, salt and pepper.

Dredge the chicken thighs in the almond flour mixture.

Place in the air fryer basket.

Cook for 30 minutes at 3500F.

Serve and enjoy!

Nutrition:
Calories: 301
Fat: 22g
Carbohydrates: 11g
Protein: 23g

Air Fried Lemon Pepper Chicken

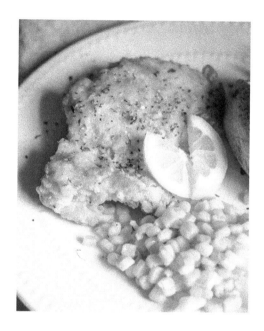

Preparation Time: 10 minutes

Cooking Time: 30 minutes

Servings: 1

Ingredients

1 chicken breast

2 lemons, sliced and rinds reserved

Salt and pepper to taste

1 teaspoon minced garlic

Directions

Preheat the air fryer at 4000F for 5 minutes.

Place all ingredients in a baking dish that will fit in the air fryer.

Place in the air fryer basket.

Cook for 20 minutes at 4000F.

Serve and enjoy!

Nutrition:
Calories: 223
Fat: 22g
Carbohydrates: 11g
Protein: 23g

Air Fried Chicken Tikkas

Preparation Time: 5 minutes

Cooking Time: 50 minutes

Servings: 4

Ingredients

1-pound chicken

1 cup coconut milk

1 bell pepper, seeded and julienned

1 teaspoon turmeric powder

1 teaspoon coriander powder

2 tablespoons olive oil

1 thumb-size ginger, grated

1 teaspoon Garam Masala

Directions

Preheat the air fryer at 3500F for 5 minutes.

Place all ingredients in a baking dish that will fit in the air fryer.

Stir to combine.

Place in the air fryer.

Cook for 50 minutes at 3500F.

Serve and enjoy!

Nutrition:

Calories: 200

Fat: 3g

Carbohydrates: 10g

Protein: 29g

Flourless Chicken Cordon Bleu

Preparation Time: 10 minutes

Cooking Time: 30 minutes

Servings: 1

Ingredients

1 chicken breast, butterflied

1 teaspoon parsley

Salt and pepper to taste

1 slice cheddar cheese

1 slice of ham

1 small egg, beaten

¼ cup almond flour

Directions

Preheat the air fryer at 3500F for 5 minutes.

Season the chicken with parsley, salt and pepper to taste.

Place the cheese and ham in the middle of the chicken and roll. Secure with toothpick.

Soak the rolled-up chicken in egg and dredge in almond flour.

Place in the air fryer.

Cook for 30 minutes at 350oF.

Nutrition:

Calories: 244

Fat: 20g

Carbohydrates: 6g

Protein: 8g

Air Fried KFC Chicken Strips

Preparation Time: 5 minutes

Cooking Time: 20 minutes

Servings: 1

Ingredients

1 chicken breast, cut into strips

1 large egg, beaten

Salt and pepper to taste

A dash of thyme

A dash of oregano

A dash of paprika

2 tablespoons unsweetened dried coconut

2 tablespoons almond flour

Directions

Preheat the air fryer at 4250F for 5 minutes

Soak the chicken in the beaten egg.

In a mixing bowl, combine the rest of the ingredients until well combined.

Dredge the chicken in the dry ingredients.

Place in the air fryer basket.

Cook for 20 minutes at 3500F.

Serve and enjoy!

Nutrition:

Calories: 423

Fat: 20g

Carbohydrates: 6g

Protein: 8g

Southern Fried Chicken Tenders

Preparation Time: 5 minutes

Cooking Time: 25 minutes

Servings: 4

Ingredients

4 chicken breasts

1 large egg

½ teaspoon cayenne pepper

½ teaspoon onion powder

½ teaspoon garlic powder

Salt and pepper to taste

¼ cup almond flour

Directions

Preheat the air fryer at 3500F for 5 minutes.

Soak the chicken in the beaten egg.

Season the chicken breasts with cayenne pepper, onion powder, garlic powder, salt and pepper.

Dredge in the almond flour.

Place in the air fryer and cook for 25 minutes at 3500F.

Serve and enjoy!

Nutrition:

Calories: 268

Fat: 20g

Carbohydrates: 6g

Protein: 8g

Easy Southern Chicken

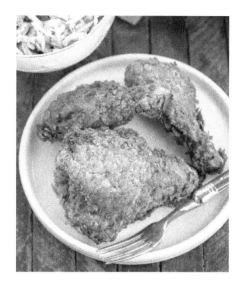

Preparation Time: 5 minutes

Cooking Time: 30 minutes

Servings: 6

Ingredients

3-pounds chicken quarters

1 teaspoon salt

1 teaspoon pepper

1 teaspoon garlic powder

1 teaspoon paprika

1 cup coconut flour

Directions

Preheat the air fryer at 350oF for 5 minutes.

Combine all ingredients in a bowl. Give a good stir.

Place ingredients in the air fryer.

Cook for 30 minutes at 350oF.

Serve and enjoy!

Nutrition:

Calories: 526
Fat: 20g
Carbohydrates: 6g
Protein: 8g

Keto Air Fryer Tandoori Chicken

Preparation Time: 2 hours

Cooking Time: 20 minutes

Servings: 4

Ingredients

1-pound chicken tenders, cut in half

½ cup coconut milk

1 tablespoon grated ginger

1 tablespoon minced garlic

¼ cup cilantro leaves, chopped

1 teaspoon turmeric

1 teaspoon Garam Masala

1 teaspoon smoked paprika

Salt and pepper to taste

Directions

Place all ingredients in a bowl and stir to coat the chicken with all ingredients.

Marinate in the fridge for 2 hours.

Preheat the air fryer at 400oF for 5 minutes.

Place the chicken pieces in the air fryer basket.

Cook for 20 minutes at 400oF.

Serve and enjoy!

Nutrition:

Calories: 255

Fat: 1g

Carbohydrates: 3g

Protein: 0g

Crispy Coconut Air Fried Chicken

Preparation Time: 5 minutes

Cooking Time: 25 minutes

Serves: 4

Ingredients

1-pound chicken tenderloins

¼ cup olive oil

¼ cup coconut flour

Salt and pepper to taste

½ teaspoon ground cumin

½ teaspoon smoked paprika

½ teaspoon garlic powder

½ teaspoon onion powder

Directions

Preheat the air fryer at 3250F for 5 minutes.

Soak the chicken tenderloins in olive oil.

Mix the rest of the ingredients and stir using your hands to combine everything.

Place the chicken pieces in the air fryer basket.

Cook for 25 minutes at 3250F.

Serve and enjoy!

Nutrition:

Calories: 353

Fat: 1g

Carbohydrates: 3g

Protein: 0g

Air Fried Chicken Drumsticks

Preparation Time: 5 minutes

Cooking Time: 30 minutes

Servings: 3

Ingredients

6 chicken drumsticks

½ cup coconut milk

½ cup almond flour

½ teaspoon salt

½ teaspoon paprika

½ teaspoon oregano

3 tablespoons melted butter

Directions

Preheat the air fryer at 250F for 5 minutes.

Soak the chicken drumsticks in coconut milk.

In a mixing bowl, combine the almond flour, salt, paprika, and oregano.

Dredge the chicken in the almond flour mixture.

Place the chicken pieces in the air fryer basket.

Air fry for 30 minutes at 3250F.

Halfway through the cooking time, give the fryer basket a shake.

Drizzle with melted butter once cooked.

Serve and enjoy!

Nutrition:

Calories: 461
Fat: 1g
Carbohydrates: 3g
Protein: 0g

Air Fried Lemon Chicken

Preparation Time: 5 minutes

Cooking Time: 30 minutes

Servings: 4

Ingredients

4 boneless chicken breasts

3 tablespoons olive oil

1 tablespoon Spanish paprika

2 tablespoons lemon juice, freshly squeezed

1 tablespoon stevia powder

 2 teaspoon minced garlic

Salt and pepper to taste

Directions

Preheat the air fryer at 3250F for 5 minutes.

Place all ingredients in a baking dish that will fit in the air fryer. Stir to combine.

Place the chicken pieces in the air fryer.

Cook for 30 minutes at 3250F.

Serve and enjoy!

Nutrition:

Calories: 296

Fat: 1g

Carbohydrates: 3g

Protein: 0g

Keto Chicken Pot Pie

Preparation Time: 5 minutes

Cooking Time: 30 minutes

Servings: 6

Ingredients

2 tablespoons butter

½ cup broccoli, chopped

¼ small onion, chopped

2 cloves of garlic, minced

¾ cup coconut milk

1 cup chicken broth

1-pound chicken, cooked, shredded

Salt and pepper to taste

4 ½ tablespoons butter, melted

1/3 cup coconut flour

4 large eggs

Directions

Preheat the air fryer at 3250F for 5 minutes.

Place 2 tablespoons butter, broccoli, onion, garlic, coconut milk, chicken broth, and chicken in a baking dish that will fit in the air fryer. Season with salt and pepper to taste.

In a mixing bowl, combine the butter, coconut flour, and eggs.

Sprinkle evenly on top of the chicken and broccoli mixture.

Place the dish in the air fryer.

Cook for 30 minutes at 3250F.

Serve and enjoy!

Nutrition:

Calories: 383
Fat: 1g
Carbohydrates: 3g
Protein: 0g

Crack Chicken

Preparation Time: 10 minutes

Cooking Time: 25 minutes

Servings: 4

Ingredients

4 chicken breasts

¼ cup olive oil

1 block cream cheese

Salt and pepper to taste

8 slices of bacon, fried and crumbled

Directions

Preheat the air fryer at 350oF for 5 minutes.

Place the chicken breasts in a baking dish that will fit in the air fryer.

Spread the olive oil, cream cheese and crumbled bacon on top of the chicken. Season with salt and pepper to taste.

Place the baking dish with the chicken and cook for 25 minutes at 3500F.

Serve and enjoy!

Nutrition:

Calories: 623

Fat: 20g

Carbohydrates: 6g

Protein: 8g

Chicken Spicata

Preparation Time: 5 minutes

Cooking Time: 35 minutes

Servings: 8

Ingredients

2 pounds chicken thighs

1 cup almond flour

4 tablespoons butter

3 tablespoons olive oil

1 medium onion, diced

½ cup chicken stock

Juice from 2 lemons, freshly squeezed

2 tablespoons capers

Salt and pepper to taste

1 large egg, beaten

Directions

Preheat the air fryer at 3250F for 5 minutes.

Combine all ingredients in a baking dish. Make sure that all lumps are removed.

Place the baking dish in the air fryer chamber.

Cook for 35 minutes at 3250F.

Serve and enjoy!

Nutrition:

Calories: 441

Fat: 54g

Carbohydrates: 4g

Protein: 30g

French Garlic Chicken

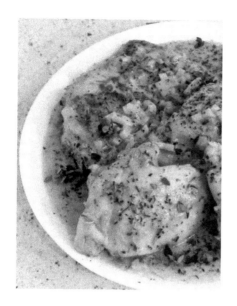

Preparation Time: 2 hours

Cooking Time: 25 minutes

Servings: 4

Ingredients

2 teaspoons herbs de Provence

2 tablespoon olive oil

1 tablespoon Dijon mustard

1 tablespoon cider vinegar

Salt and pepper to taste

1-pound chicken thighs

Directions

Place all ingredients in a Ziploc bag.

Marinate in the fridge for at least 2 hours.

Preheat the air fryer at 3500F for 5 minutes.

Place the chicken in the fryer basket.

Cook for 25 minutes at 3500F.

Serve and enjoy!

Nutrition:

Calories: 175

Fat: 1g

Carbohydrates: 3g

Protein: 0g

Meat

Juicy Pork Chops

Preparation Time: 10 minutes

Cooking Time: 16 minutes

Servings: 4

Ingredients:

4 pork chops, boneless

2 tsp olive oil

½ tsp celery seed

½ tsp parsley

½ tsp granulated onion

½ tsp granulated garlic

¼ tsp sugar

½ tsp salt

Directions:

In a small bowl, mix together oil, celery seed, parsley, granulated onion, granulated garlic, sugar, and salt.

Rub seasoning mixture all over the pork chops.

Place pork chops on the air fryer oven pan and cook at 350 F for 8 minutes.

Turn pork chops to other side and cook for 8 minutes more.

Serve and enjoy.

Nutrition:
Calories 279
Fat 22.3 g
Carbohydrates 0.6 g
Sugar 0.3 g
Protein 18.1 g
Cholesterol 69 mg

Crispy Meatballs

Preparation Time: 10 minutes

Cooking Time: 12 minutes

Servings: 8

Ingredients:

1 lb. ground pork

1 lb. ground beef

1 tbsp Worcestershire sauce

½ cup feta cheese, crumbled

½ cup breadcrumbs

2 eggs, lightly beaten

¼ cup fresh parsley, chopped

1 tbsp garlic, minced

1 onion, chopped

¼ tsp pepper

1 tsp salt

Directions:

Add all ingredients into the mixing bowl and mix until well combined.

Spray air fryer oven tray pan with cooking spray.

Make small balls from meat mixture and arrange on a pan and air fry t 400 F for 10-12 minutes.

Serve and enjoy.

Nutrition:

Calories 263

Fat 9 g

Carbohydrates 7.5 g

Sugar 1.9 g

Protein 35.9 g

Cholesterol 141 mg

Flavorful Steak

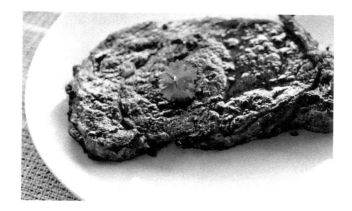

Preparation Time: 10 minutes

Cooking Time: 18 minutes

Servings: 2

Ingredients:

2 steaks, rinsed and pat dry

½ tsp garlic powder

1 tsp olive oil

Pepper

Salt

Directions:

Rub steaks with olive oil and season with garlic powder, pepper, and salt.

Preheat the instant vortex air fryer oven to 400 F.

Place steaks on air fryer oven pan and air fry for 10-18 minutes. Turn halfway through.

Serve and enjoy.

Nutrition:

Calories 361

Fat 10.9 g

Carbohydrates 0.5 g

Sugar 0.2 g

Protein 61.6 g

Cholesterol 153 mg

Lemon Garlic Lamb Chops

Preparation Time: 10 minutes

Cooking Time: 6 minutes

Servings: 6

Ingredients:

6 lamb loin chops

2 tbsp fresh lemon juice

1 ½ tbsp lemon zest

1 tbsp dried rosemary

1 tbsp olive oil

1 tbsp garlic, minced

Pepper

Salt

Directions:

Add lamb chops in a mixing bowl.

Add remaining ingredients on top of lamb chops and coat well.

Arrange lamb chops on air fryer oven tray and air fry at 400 F for 3 minutes.

Turn lamb chops to another side and air fry for 3 minutes more.

Serve and enjoy.

Nutrition:

Calories 69

Fat 6 g

Carbohydrates 1.2 g

Sugar 0.2 g

Protein 3 g

Cholesterol 0 mg

Honey Mustard Pork Tenderloin

Preparation Time: 10 minutes

Cooking Time: 26 minutes

Servings: 4

Ingredients:

1 lb. pork tenderloin

1 tsp sriracha sauce

1 tbsp garlic, minced

2 tbsp soy sauce

1 ½ tbsp honey

¾ tbsp Dijon mustard

1 tbsp mustard

Directions:

Add sriracha sauce, garlic, soy sauce, honey, Dijon mustard, and mustard into the large zip-lock bag and mix well.

Add pork tenderloin into the bag. Seal bag and place in the refrigerator for overnight.

Preheat the instant vortex air fryer oven to 380 F.

Spray instant vortex air fryer tray with cooking spray then place marinated pork tenderloin on a tray and air fry for 26 minutes. Turn pork tenderloin after every 5 minutes.

Slice and serve.

Nutrition:
Calories 195
Fat 4.1 g
Carbohydrates 8 g
Sugar 6.7 g
Protein 30.5 g
Cholesterol 83 mg

Easy Rosemary Lamb Chops

Preparation Time: 10 minutes

Cooking Time: 6 minutes

Servings: 4

Ingredients:

4 lamb chops

2 tbsp dried rosemary

¼ cup fresh lemon juice

Pepper

Salt

Directions:

In a small bowl, mix together lemon juice, rosemary, pepper, and salt.

Brush lemon juice rosemary mixture over lamb chops.

Place lamb chops on air fryer oven tray and air fry at 400 F for 3 minutes.

Turn lamb chops to the other side and cook for 3 minutes more.

Serve and enjoy.

Nutrition:

Calories 267

Fat 21.7 g

Carbohydrates 1.4 g

Sugar 0.3 g

Protein 16.9 g

Cholesterol 0 mg

BBQ Pork Ribs

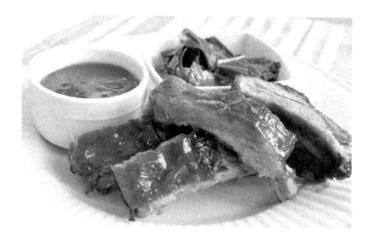

Preparation Time: 10 minutes

Cooking Time: 12 minutes

Servings: 6

Ingredients:

1 slab baby back pork ribs, cut into pieces

½ cup BBQ sauce

½ tsp paprika

Salt

Directions:

Add pork ribs in a mixing bowl.

Add BBQ sauce, paprika, and salt over pork ribs and coat well and set aside for 30 minutes.

Preheat the instant vortex air fryer oven to 350 F.

Arrange marinated pork ribs on instant vortex air fryer oven pan and cook for 10-12 minutes. Turn halfway through.

Serve and enjoy.

Nutrition:
Calories 145
Fat 7 g
Carbohydrates 10 g
Sugar 7 g
Protein 9 g
Cholesterol 30 mg

Juicy Steak Bites

Preparation Time: 10 minutes

Cooking Time: 9 minutes

Servings: 4

Ingredients:

1 lb. sirloin steak, cut into bite-size pieces

1 tbsp steak seasoning

1 tbsp olive oil

Pepper

Salt

Directions:

Preheat the instant vortex air fryer oven to 390 F.

Add steak pieces into the large mixing bowl. Add steak seasoning, oil, pepper, and salt over steak pieces and toss until well coated.

Transfer steak pieces on instant vortex air fryer pan and air fry for 5 minutes.

Turn steak pieces to the other side and cook for 4 minutes more.

Serve and enjoy.

Nutrition:
Calories 241
Fat 10.6 g
Carbohydrates 0 g
Sugar 0 g
Protein 34.4 g
Cholesterol 101 mg

Greek Lamb Chops

Preparation Time: 10 minutes

Cooking Time: 10 minutes

Servings: 4

Ingredients:

2 lbs. lamb chops

2 tsp garlic, minced

1 ½ tsp dried oregano

¼ cup fresh lemon juice

¼ cup olive oil

½ tsp pepper

1 tsp salt

Directions:

Add lamb chops in a mixing bowl. Add remaining ingredients over the lamb chops and coat well.

Arrange lamb chops on the air fryer oven tray and cook at 400 F for 5 minutes.

Turn lamb chops and cook for 5 minutes more.

Serve and enjoy.

Nutrition:

Calories 538

Fat 29.4 g

Carbohydrates 1.3 g

Sugar 0.4 g

Protein 64 g

Cholesterol 204 mg

Easy Beef Roast

Preparation Time: 10 minutes

Cooking Time: 45 minutes

Servings: 6

Ingredients:

2 ½ lbs. beef roast

2 tbsp Italian seasoning

Directions:

Arrange roast on the rotisserie spite.

Rub roast with Italian seasoning then insert into the instant vortex air fryer oven.

Air fry at 350 F for 45 minutes or until the internal temperature of the roast reaches to 145 F.

Slice and serve.

Nutrition:

Calories 365 ,Fat 13.2 g Carbohydrates 0.5 g

Sugar 0.4 g, Protein 57.4 g, Cholesterol 172 mg

Herb Butter Rib-eye Steak

Preparation Time: 10 minutes

Cooking Time: 14 minutes

Servings: 4

Ingredients:

2 lbs. rib eye steak, bone-in

1 tsp fresh rosemary, chopped

1 tsp fresh thyme, chopped

1 tsp fresh chives, chopped

2 tsp fresh parsley, chopped

1 tsp garlic, minced

¼ cup butter softened

Pepper

Salt

Directions:

In a small bowl, combine together butter and herbs.

Rub herb butter on rib-eye steak and place it in the refrigerator for 30 minutes.

Place marinated steak on instant vortex air fryer oven pan and cook at 400 F for 12-14 minutes.

Serve and enjoy.

Nutrition:

Calories 416

Fat 36.7 g

Carbohydrates 0.7 g

Sugar 0 g

Protein 20.3 g

Cholesterol 106 mg

BBQ Pork Chops

Preparation Time: 10 minutes

Cooking Time: 7 minutes

Servings: 4

Ingredients:

4 pork chops

For rub:

½ tsp allspice

½ tsp dry mustard

1 tsp ground cumin

1 tsp garlic powder

½ tsp chili powder

½ tsp paprika

1 tbsp brown sugar

1 tsp salt

Directions:

In a small bowl, mix together all rub ingredients and rub all over pork chops.

Arrange pork chops on air fryer tray and air fry at 400 F for 5.

Turn pork chops to other side and air fry for 2 minutes more.

Serve and enjoy.

Nutrition:

Calories 273

Fat 20.2 g

Carbohydrates 3.4 g

Sugar 2.4 g

Protein 18.4 g

Cholesterol 69 mg

Marinated Pork Chops

Preparation Time: 10 minutes

Cooking Time: 30 minutes

Servings: 2

Ingredients:

2 pork chops, boneless

1 tsp garlic powder

½ cup flour

1 cup buttermilk

Pepper

Salt

Directions:

Add pork chops and buttermilk in a zip-lock bag. Seal bag and place in the refrigerator for overnight.

In another zip-lock bag add flour, garlic powder, pepper, and salt.

Remove marinated pork chops from buttermilk and add in flour mixture and shake until well coated.

Preheat the instant vortex air fryer oven to 380 F.

Spray air fryer tray with cooking spray.

Arrange pork chops on a tray and air fryer for 28-30 minutes. Turn pork chops after 18 minutes.

Serve and enjoy.

Nutrition:
Calories 424
Fat 21.3 g
Carbohydrates 30.8 g
Sugar 6.3 g
Protein 25.5 g
Cholesterol 74 mg

Chimichurri Sauce and Skirt Steak

Preparation Time: 30 minutes

Cooking Time: 10 minutes

Servings: 4

Ingredients:

16 ounces skirt steak

Chimichurri Sauce

1 cup parsley, chopped

¼ cup mint, chopped

2 tablespoons oregano, chopped

3 garlic cloves, chopped

1 teaspoon crushed red pepper

1 tablespoon cumin, grounded

1 teaspoon cayenne pepper

2 teaspoons smoked paprika

1 teaspoon salt

¼ teaspoon pepper

¾ cup olive oil

3 tablespoons red wine vinegar

Directions:

Take a bowl and mix all of the Ingredients: listed under Chimichurri section and mix them well

Cut the steak into 2 pieces of 8-ounce portions

Take a re-sealable bag and add ¼ cup of Chimichurri alongside the steak pieces and shake them to ensure that steak is coated well

Allow it to chill in your fridge for 2-24 hours

Remove the steak from the fridge 30 minutes prior to cooking

Pre-heat your Fryer to 390-degree Fahrenheit

Transfer the steak to your Fryer and cook for about 8-10 minutes if you are looking for a medium-rare finish

Garnish with 2 tablespoon of Chimichurri sauce and enjoy!

Nutrition:

Calories: 244

Fat: 18g

Carbohydrates: 7g

Protein: 13g

Beef and Tomato Balls

Preparation Time: 10 minutes

Cooking Time: 5 minutes

Servings: 4

Ingredients:

1 small onion, chopped

¾ pounds ground beef

1 tablespoon fresh parsley, chopped

½ tablespoon fresh thyme leaves, chopped

1 whole egg

3 tablespoons almond meal

Salt and pepper to taste

Directions:

Chop onion and keep them on the side

Take a bowl and add listed Ingredients: mix well (including onions)

Make 12 balls

Pre-heat your Air Fryer to 390 degrees F, transfer balls to the fryer

Cook for 8 minutes (in batches if needed) and transfer the balls to oven

Add tomatoes sauce and drown the balls

Transfer the dish to your Air Fryer and cook for 5 minutes at 300 degrees F

Stir and serve

Enjoy!

Nutrition:

Calories: 257

Fat: 18g

Carbohydrates: 6g

Protein: 15g

Herbed Up Roast Beef

Preparation Time: 15 minutes

Cooking Time: 12 minutes

Servings: 4

Ingredients:

2 teaspoons olive oil

4-pound top round roast beef

1 teaspoon salt

¼ teaspoon fresh ground black pepper

1 teaspoon dried thyme

½ teaspoon rosemary, chopped

3 pounds red potatoes, halved

Olive oil, fresh ground black pepper and salt to taste

Directions:

Pre-heat your Air Fryer to 360-degree F

Rub olive oil all over the beef

Take a bowl and add rosemary, thyme, salt and pepper

Mix well

Season the beef with the mixture and transfer the meat to your Fryer

Cook for 20 minutes

Add potatoes alongside some pepper and oil

Turn the roast alongside and add the potatoes to the basket

Cook for 20 minutes

Make sure to rotate the mixture from time to time

Cook until you have reached your desired temperature (130F for Rare, 140F for Medium and 160F for Well Done)

Once done, allow the meat to cool for 10 minutes

Pre-heat your Air Fryer to 400-degree Fahrenheit and keep cooking the potatoes for 10 minutes

Serve with the potatoes with the beef and enjoy!

Nutrition:

Calories: 523

Fat: 63g

Carbohydrates: 4g

Protein: 37g

Conclusion

When you are on a diet trying to lose weight or manage a condition, you will be strictly confined to follow an eating plan. Such plans often place numerous demands on individuals: food may need to be boiled, other foods are forbidden, permitting you only to eat small portions and so on.

On the other hand, a lifestyle such as the Mediterranean diet is entirely stress-free. It is easy to follow because there are almost no restrictions. There is no time limit on the Mediterranean diet because it is more of a lifestyle than a diet. You do not need to stop at some point but carry on for the rest of your life. The foods that you eat under the Mediterranean model include unrefined cereals, white meats, and the occasional dairy products.

The Mediterranean lifestyle, unlike other diets, also requires you to engage with family and friends and share meals together. It has been noted that communities around the Mediterranean spend between one and two hours enjoying their meals. This kind of bonding between family members or friends helps bring people closer together, which helps foster closer bonds hence fewer cases of depression, loneliness, or stress, all of which are precursors to chronic diseases.

You will achieve many benefits using the Instant Pot Pressure Cooker. These are just a few instances you will discover in your Mediterranean-style recipes:

Pressure cooking means that you can (on average) cook meals 75% faster than boiling/braising on the stovetop or baking and roasting in a conventional oven.

This is especially helpful for vegan meals that entail the use of dried beans, legumes, and pulses. Instead of pre-soaking these ingredients for hours before use, you can pour them directly into the Instant Pot, add water, and pressure cook these for several minutes. However, always follow your recipe carefully since they have been tested for accuracy.

Nutrients are preserved. You can use your pressure-cooking techniques using the Instant Pot to ensure the heat is evenly and quickly distributed. It is not essential to immerse the food into the water. You will provide plenty of water in the cooker for efficient steaming. You will also be saving the essential vitamins and minerals. The food won't become oxidized by the exposure of air or heat. Enjoy those fresh green veggies with their natural and vibrant colors.

The cooking elements help keep the foods fully sealed, so the steam and aromas don't linger throughout your entire home. That is a plus, especially for items such as cabbage, which throws out a distinctive smell.

You will find that beans and whole grains will have a softer texture and will have an improved taste. The meal will be cooked consistently since the Instant Pot provides even heat distribution.

You'll also save tons of time and money. You will be using much less water, and the pot is fully insulated, making it more energy-efficient when compared to boiling or steaming your foods on the stovetop. It is also less expensive than using a microwave, not to mention how much more flavorful the food will be when prepared in the Instant Pot cooker.

You can delay the cooking of your food items so you can plan ahead of time. You won't need to stand around as you await your meal. You can reduce the cooking time by reducing the 'hands-on' time. Just leave for work or a day of activities, and you will come home to a special treat.

In a nutshell, the Instant Pot is:

Easy To Use Healthy recipes for the entire family are provided.

You can make authentic one-pot recipes in your Instant Pot.

If you forget to switch on your slow cooker, you can make any meal done in a few minutes in your Instant Pot.

You can securely and smoothly cook meat from frozen.

It's a laid-back way to cook. You don't have to watch a pan on the stove or a pot in the oven.

The pressure cooking procedure develops delicious flavors swiftly.

CPSIA information can be obtained
at www.ICGtesting.com
Printed in the USA
LVHW080326200421
684918LV00019B/1741